ENDOMETRIOSIS DIET PLAN FOR SENIORS

Unlocking Comfort and Health in Your Golden Years

Lizzy James

TABLE OF CONTENTS

INTRODUCTION

Welcome to a journey of empowerment, health, and well-being tailored specifically for the vibrant senior women navigating the complexities of endometriosis. As the golden years unfold, embracing life with vitality becomes paramount, and yet, the presence of endometriosis can cast shadows on this beautiful chapter. But fear not, for this guide is a beacon of hope—an exploration into the transformative power of nutrition.

Endometriosis, a condition that affects millions of women worldwide, doesn't exempt our wise and wonderful seniors. It brings with it unique challenges that demand a nuanced approach to healthcare. This is where the "Endometriosis Diet Plan for Seniors" steps in—a comprehensive roadmap designed not just to manage symptoms but to empower you to reclaim control over your health.

In the chapters that follow, we delve into the intricate dance between nutrition, inflammation, and hormonal balance. We unravel the mysteries of foods that can soothe, nourish, and fortify your body against the challenges of endometriosis. This isn't just a diet plan; it's a lifestyle compass guiding you toward choices that resonate with your unique needs, allowing you to flourish in your later years.

So, whether you're a senior woman seeking relief, a caregiver supporting a loved one, or a health enthusiast curious about the intersection of nutrition and endometriosis in the golden years, this guide is your ally. Let's embark on a journey where the right foods become your allies, and each bite contributes to a life rich in joy, wellness, and resilience. The "Endometriosis Diet Plan for Seniors" is not just a guide; it's a celebration of the strength within you, embracing the beauty of aging with grace and vitality.

CHAPTER ONE

INTRODUCTION

Understanding Endometriosis in Seniors

Understanding endometriosis in the elderly requires a comprehensive investigation of the illness in relation to aging. The main procedures involved are as follows:

1. Symptom Awareness in Seniors:

Anomalies in Signs Identification: Elderly people may have distinct endometriosis symptoms that are not present in younger people. Urinary symptoms, bowel behavior changes, and pelvic pain are a few examples of these. Understanding these symptoms is essential for prompt diagnosis and treatment.

Difference from conditions connected to age: Elderly people frequently struggle with a range of age-related health problems. Accurate diagnosis and focused care for endometriosis require an understanding of how its symptoms present and differ from those of other common age-related illnesses.

2. Impact on Life Quality:

Aspects related to the body and the mind: Seniors with endometriosis may experience substantial reductions in quality of life. There may be issues with weariness, emotional stability, and chronic discomfort. Investigating the relationship between mental and physical health facilitates the development of comprehensive plans to enhance general wellbeing.

Implications for society: It's critical to comprehend how endometriosis affects social facets of a senior's life, including relationships and everyday activities. It entails identifying the possible obstacles and figuring out how to lessen their impact on engagement and social ties.

3. Aging Body Considerations:

Changes in Hormones: As they age, seniors naturally go through hormonal changes. Customizing successful therapies requires an understanding of how these alterations interact with endometriosis. This entails investigating the potential effects of menopausal hormone variations on the development and manifestation of endometriosis.

Concurrent medical conditions: Elderly people frequently handle several medical concerns at once. Understanding the interplay between endometriosis and other age-related health problems is essential to delivering all-encompassing care.

4. Diagnostic Difficulties:

Diagnostic Nuances linked to Age: Due to age-related changes in symptom presentation, diagnosing endometriosis in seniors can be difficult. It is critical to recognize these subtleties and use age-appropriate diagnostic techniques, like imaging and less invasive treatments.

Barriers to communication: Accurate diagnosis depends on seniors and healthcare professionals having effective communication. Part of the process involves addressing potential hurdles to communication, such as generational differences or the stigma associated with reproductive health among the elderly.

Importance of Nutrition in Managing Endometriosis

Managing endometriosis through nutrition is a crucial component of comprehensive care. Endometriosis symptoms and progression are significantly influenced by nutrition, which provides both short-term symptom relief and long-term treatment. This article explores the importance of nutrition in the treatment of endometriosis.

1. Control of Inflammation:

Anti-inflammatory Foods: Some foods have anti-inflammatory qualities that can help reduce the ongoing inflammation linked to endometriosis. Stressing the importance of eating a diet high in fruits, vegetables, whole grains, and fatty fish will help to lower inflammation, which in turn helps to lessen pain and suffering.

2. Environmental Equilibrium:

Effect on Hormones: Hormonal equilibrium is significantly impacted by nutrition. Hormonal variations, especially those related to estrogen, have an impact on endometriosis. A balanced diet has the ability to reduce symptoms related to hormone imbalances by assisting in the regulation of hormone levels.

3. Support for the Immune System:

Foods High in Nutrients: A diet rich in nutrients helps the immune system work as a whole. Ensuring sufficient consumption of vitamins, minerals, and antioxidants can improve the immune response and aid in the management of endometriosis, as the condition is caused by the immune system reacting to misplaced endometrial tissue.

4. Body Mass Index (BMI): Weight Management: Keeping a healthy weight is essential for endometriosis management. Higher estrogen levels can be a contributing factor to excess body fat, which exacerbates symptoms. A healthy BMI is largely attained and maintained through nutrition, which also has a good impact on hormone balance and general wellbeing.

5. Digestive Comfort and Gut Health:

Foods High in Fiber: Consuming dietary fiber helps maintain gut health and regular bowel movements, which is especially advantageous for those who have endometriosis. A healthy digestive system lessens bloating and discomfort, which benefits people's general wellbeing.

6. Status of Energy and Fatigue:

Equilibrated Macronutrients: A balanced diet that includes carbohydrates, proteins, and fats will provide you with long-lasting energy. This is essential for controlling the exhaustion that endometriosis patients frequently experience, enabling them to lead active lives and participate in everyday activities.

7. Mind-Body Connection:

Nourishment for Stress Reduction: Some foods, such as those high in omega-3 fatty acids, have been shown to have a good effect on mental health. Because stress can worsen the symptoms of endometriosis, managing stress through nutrition is crucial. Including foods that reduce stress contributes to the mind-body connection, which is essential for general wellbeing.

8. Personalized Nutrition Plans:

Individualized Approaches: Individualized nutrition programs can be created for those with endometriosis, taking into account their specific needs. Nutrition interventions that take into account variables such as dietary sensitivity, preference, and cultural influences are guaranteed to be both successful and long-lasting for long-term care.

Overview of the Endometriosis Diet Plan

The Endometriosis Diet Plan is a comprehensive and personalized approach to nutrition aimed at managing the symptoms and improving the quality of life for individuals dealing with endometriosis. It goes beyond being just a list of dietary dos and don'ts; rather, it is a dynamic strategy that considers the unique needs and experiences of each individual.

1. Understanding Individual Needs:

Personalized Assessment: The diet plan begins with a thorough assessment of the individual's health history, symptoms, and lifestyle. This personalized approach ensures that the diet plan is tailored to meet the specific needs and challenges of the person with endometriosis.

2. Anti-Inflammatory Emphasis:

Incorporating Anti-Inflammatory Foods: Given that inflammation is a central component of endometriosis, the diet plan focuses on incorporating foods with anti-inflammatory properties. This includes a variety of fruits, vegetables, whole grains, and fatty fish rich in omega-3 fatty acids, which can help alleviate inflammation and associated symptoms.

3. Hormone-Balancing Strategies:

Supporting Hormonal Balance: Hormonal fluctuations, particularly estrogen levels, play a role in endometriosis. The diet plan includes foods that support hormonal balance, such as those with phytoestrogens and nutrients that aid in estrogen metabolism. This strategic approach aims to address hormonal imbalances associated with endometriosis.

4. Emphasis on Nutrient Density:

Nutrient-Rich Foods: The plan encourages the consumption of nutrient-dense foods to provide essential vitamins and minerals. This not only supports overall health but also boosts the immune system, contributing to the body's ability to manage the challenges posed by endometriosis.

5. Balanced Macronutrients:

Proper Balance of Carbohydrates, Proteins, and Fats: Ensuring a balanced intake of macronutrients is essential for sustained energy levels and overall well-being. The diet plan includes a variety of foods that provide the necessary balance, promote energy, and help manage fatigue often associated with endometriosis.

6. Gut Health Optimization:

Fiber and Probiotic-Rich Foods: A healthy gut is crucial for individuals with endometriosis. The diet plan includes foods rich in fiber to support digestive health and incorporates probiotic-rich foods to promote a balanced gut microbiome, which may positively impact symptoms.

7. Mindful Eating and Stress Management:

Stress-Reducing Nutrition: Recognizing the mind-body connection, the diet plan integrates foods that can help manage stress. Stress reduction is particularly important since stress can exacerbate endometriosis symptoms. Mindful eating practices are also encouraged to foster a positive relationship with food.

8. Long-Term Sustainability:

Lifestyle Integration: The Endometriosis Diet Plan is designed to be sustainable in the long term. It takes into account the practical aspects of daily life, providing guidance on meal planning, preparation, and making informed choices in various social and cultural contexts.

CHAPTER TWO

BASICS OF ENDOMETRIOSIS

What is Endometriosis?

The presence and proliferation of tissue outside the uterus that resembles the endometrium—the lining of the uterus—is a persistent medical disorder known as endometriosis. This illness can result in a variety of symptoms and consequences and mainly affects people with reproductive anatomy, usually women. Now let's explore the many facets of endometriosis:

1. Tissue Growth Abnormality:

Pathophysiology: Endometrial-like tissue grows outside the uterus in endometriosis. The lining of the pelvic cavity, the uterus' exterior, the ovaries, fallopian tubes, and, in rare instances, distant organs including the lungs can all develop endometrial implants.

2. Indications:

Pelvic Pain: This is the most prevalent symptom, and its severity may not always be directly related to the severity of the ailment.

Irregular Menstruation: Those who have endometriosis frequently have heavy or irregular menstrual cycles.

Painful Intercourse: A common complaint is pain experienced during or following sex.

Intestinal Ailments: Digestion problems and pain during bowel movements, particularly during menstruation, might be brought on by endometriosis.

3. Diagnosis:

Clinical Assessment: A thorough medical history that covers symptoms and how they affect day-to-day functioning is typically the first step in making a diagnosis.

Imaging Studies: Endometrial implants can be seen with ultrasound and magnetic resonance imaging (MRI).

Laparoscopy: Laparoscopy, a minimally invasive surgical procedure, is the gold standard for diagnosis. An endometrial implant can be directly visualized and treated by a surgeon during this surgery, if needed.

4. Risk Factors:

Age and Menstrual History: Endometriosis usually manifests during the reproductive years, and those who begin menstruation early may be at a higher risk.

Family History: People who have a close family member who has endometriosis, like a mother or sister, may be more susceptible.

Uterine Abnormalities: Endometriosis can arise as a result of anatomical abnormalities that prevent the menstrual blood flow from occurring normally.

5. A Effect on Fertility: Decreased Fertility: One of the main causes of infertility in women is endometriosis. It impairs fertility through a variety of methods, such as inflammation, deformity of the reproductive organs, and the development of an adverse environment for conception.

6. Management and Treatment:

Pain Management: Using pharmaceuticals such as nonsteroidal anti-inflammatory drugs (NSAIDs) and hormonal treatments, pain reduction is the main goal of treatment.

Surgical Procedures: Laparoscopic surgery is frequently utilized for endometrial implant removal as well as diagnostics. A hysterectomy, or the removal of the uterus, may be considered in extreme circumstances.

Endocrine Supplements: The goal of several hormonal therapies, including hormonal IUDs, GnRH agonists, and birth control tablets, is to inhibit menstruation and slow the formation of endometrial tissue.

7. Quality of Life Aspects:

Managing Chronic Conditions: Since endometriosis is a chronic illness, long-term care is necessary. A mix of lifestyle, surgical, and medicinal therapies may be used to achieve this.

Emotional Effect: Fertility issues and chronic discomfort can have a major psychological impact. Comprehensive management frequently includes supportive care, such as counseling and support groups.

8. Continuous Research:

Investigation of Root Causes: There is still much to learn about the precise cause of endometriosis. Investigations on the genetic, hormonal, and environmental elements influencing its development are still ongoing.

9. Creative Solutions: Novel therapeutic techniques and treatments, such as immunotherapies and targeted drugs, are being studied in ongoing research.

Symptoms in Senior Women

Endometriosis affects women of all ages, including seniors, despite the fact that it is typically linked to younger women who are fertile. These are ten to fifteen signs that older women may have endometriosis:

1. Pelvic Pain: This refers to recurrent or persistent pelvic pain that might not be the same as regular menstrual cramps.

2. Lower Back Pain: Lower back pain that is persistent or recurrent and is not only caused by musculoskeletal problems

3. Painful Menstruation: Menstrual cycles marked by excruciating pain, cramps, or other discomfort

4. Irregular Menstruation: Variations in the menstrual cycles' regularity or intensity

5. Painful Intercourse: Pain or discomfort experienced during sex, especially when being penetrated.

6. Symptoms Related to the Stomach: signs including bloating, constipation, diarrhea, or pain in the abdomen, particularly during menstruation.

7. Urinary issues: These include frequent urination, urgency, or pain during the process that does not seem to be related to an infection of the urinary system.\

8. Fatigue: extended tiredness that cannot be fully attributed to another medical issue.

9. Bleeding Between Periods: In the interim between menstrual cycles, there may be spotting or bleeding.

10. Difficult Bowel Movements: Pain or discomfort **during** the menstrual cycle, particularly during the bowel movements.

11. Pelvic discomfort: a sensation of heaviness or general discomfort in the pelvic area.

12. Painful Ovulation: This might be a clear sign of endometriosis, discomfort, or pain during ovulation.

13. Sorrowful Scarring: As endometriosis can impact different pelvic structures, pain or discomfort associated with prior surgeries or scarring

14. Trouble Emptying the Bladder or Bowels: Trouble emptying the bladder or bowels entirely, probably because endometrial tissue is present.

15. Emotional Impact: Changes in mood, anxiety, or depression associated with the long-term nature of the symptoms and how they affect day-to-day functioning

Impact on Quality of Life

Endometriosis can have a profound impact on the quality of life for individuals affected by this condition. The symptoms and challenges associated with endometriosis often extend beyond physical discomfort, influencing various aspects of daily life and overall well-being. Here's an exploration of the impact on quality of life:

1. Chronic Pain:

Physical Discomfort: Persistent pelvic pain, often accompanied by menstruation, can significantly impact one's ability to engage in daily activities, work, and enjoy life without discomfort.

2. Emotional Well-being:

Mood Disturbances: The chronic nature of endometriosis and the associated pain can lead to mood swings, anxiety, and depression, affecting emotional stability and overall mental health.

3. Social Relationships:

Intimacy Issues: Painful intercourse and ongoing discomfort may strain intimate relationships, potentially affecting both physical and emotional intimacy.

Social Isolation: Coping with chronic pain and unpredictable symptoms may lead to social withdrawal or a sense of isolation, impacting social activities and relationships.

4. Occupational Impact:

Work Productivity: Chronic pain and associated symptoms can interfere with work productivity and attendance, potentially leading to professional challenges and career limitations.

5. Fertility Concerns:

Emotional Strain: The potential impact of endometriosis on fertility can cause emotional distress and strain for individuals or couples aspiring to build a family.

6. Fatigue and Energy Levels:

Daily Functioning: Persistent fatigue, common in endometriosis, can limit energy levels, affecting the ability to perform everyday tasks and engage in physical activities.

7. Financial Strain:

Healthcare Costs: Managing endometriosis often involves medical treatments, surgeries, and ongoing healthcare expenses, leading to financial burdens for individuals and their families.

8. Coping Mechanisms:

Adaptation and Coping: Constantly managing pain and navigating the challenges of endometriosis may necessitate the development of coping mechanisms, impacting one's lifestyle and daily routine.

9. Diagnostic Delays and Frustration:

Frustration with Diagnosis: The diagnostic journey for endometriosis can be lengthy and frustrating. Delays in obtaining a diagnosis may contribute to ongoing physical and emotional distress.

10. Impact on Sleep:

Sleep Disturbances: Chronic pain and discomfort can interfere with sleep quality, leading to sleep disturbances and contributing to overall fatigue and irritability.

11. Healthcare Utilization:

Frequent Medical Visits: The need for regular medical appointments, treatments, and interventions can lead to increased healthcare utilization and potential disruptions to daily life.

12. Personal Empowerment:

Advocacy and Education: Living with endometriosis often involves becoming an advocate for one's health, educating oneself about the condition, and actively participating in treatment decisions.

CHAPTER THREE

NUTRITIONAL FOUNDATIONS

Importance of a Balanced Diet

A balanced diet is essential for maintaining optimal health and well-being across all stages of life. It involves consuming a variety of foods in appropriate proportions to provide the body with the necessary nutrients for growth, development, and daily functioning. Here are several key reasons highlighting the importance of a balanced diet:

1. Nutrient Intake:

Essential Nutrients: A balanced diet ensures the intake of essential nutrients, including proteins, carbohydrates, fats, vitamins, and minerals, that are crucial for the body's proper functioning.

2. Energy for Daily Activities:

Optimal Energy Levels: Carbohydrates, fats, and proteins from a balanced diet serve as energy sources, providing the fuel needed for daily activities, work, and exercise.

3. Maintaining a Healthy Weight:

Weight Management: A balanced diet helps in achieving and maintaining a healthy weight by providing the right balance of calories and nutrients. This is essential for preventing both undernutrition and obesity-related health issues.

4. Supporting Growth and Development:

Vital for Children and Adolescents: Children and adolescents require a balanced diet to support growth, development, and the formation of healthy tissues, organs, and bones.

5. Disease Prevention:

Reducing the Risk of Chronic Diseases: A diet rich in fruits, vegetables, whole grains, and lean proteins has been associated with a lower risk of chronic diseases such as heart disease, diabetes, and certain types of cancer.

6. Optimal Organ Function:

Supporting Organ Health: Nutrient-rich foods contribute to the proper functioning of vital organs such as the heart, kidneys, liver, and brain, promoting overall health.

7. Bone Health:

Calcium and Vitamin D: Adequate intake of calcium and vitamin D, found in dairy products and other foods, is crucial for maintaining strong and healthy bones.

8. Digestive Health:

Fiber Intake: A balanced diet with sufficient fiber promotes healthy digestion, prevents constipation, and supports a diverse and beneficial gut microbiome.

9. Immune System Support:

Vitamins and Minerals: Essential vitamins and minerals, including vitamin C, vitamin A, zinc, and selenium, play a crucial role in supporting the immune system and defending the body against infections.

10. Heart Health:

Healthy Fats: Including sources of healthy fats, such as omega-3 fatty acids found in fish, can contribute to heart health by lowering cholesterol levels and reducing the risk of cardiovascular diseases.

11. Blood Sugar Regulation:

Balanced Blood Sugar Levels: A balanced diet helps regulate blood sugar levels, reducing the risk of insulin resistance and type 2 diabetes.

12. Mental Health:

Brain Function: Nutrient-rich foods, including those with omega-3 fatty acids, are important for cognitive function and may contribute to mental well-being.

13. Recovery and Healing:

Tissue Repair: After injury or illness, a balanced diet provides the necessary nutrients for tissue repair, recovery, and healing.

Essential Nutrients for Senior Women

As individuals age, their nutritional needs may change, and ensuring the intake of essential nutrients becomes crucial for maintaining health and well-being. Senior women, in particular, may have specific requirements to address age-related changes. Here are some essential nutrients that are important for senior women:

1. Calcium:

Importance: Essential for maintaining bone health and preventing osteoporosis.

Sources: dairy products, leafy green vegetables, fortified plant-based milk, and fish with edible bones.

2. Vitamin D:

Importance: Facilitates calcium absorption, promoting bone health and immune function.

Sources: Sunlight exposure, fatty fish, fortified dairy or plant-based milk, and supplements if needed.

3. Vitamin B12:

Importance: It supports nerve function, red blood cell production, and helps prevent anemia.

Sources: Meat, fish, dairy products, and fortified foods; supplementation may be necessary for those with absorption issues.

4. Fiber:

Importance: It aids digestion, helps prevent constipation, and supports heart health.

Sources: Whole grains, fruits, vegetables, legumes, and nuts

5. Potassium:

Importance: It maintains fluid balance, supports heart health, and helps regulate blood pressure.

***Sources:** bananas, oranges, potatoes, tomatoes, leafy greens, and low-fat dairy products.

6. Omega-3 Fatty Acids:

Importance: It supports heart health and cognitive function and may have anti-inflammatory effects.

Sources: Fatty fish (salmon, trout, mackerel), flaxseeds, chia seeds, and walnuts

7. Magnesium:

Importance: Supports bone health and muscle function and may help regulate blood pressure.

Sources: Nuts, seeds, whole grains, leafy green vegetables, and legumes

8. Iron:

Importance: Important for preventing anemia and supporting energy levels.

Sources: Lean meats, poultry, fish, fortified cereals, and dark leafy greens

9. Zinc:

Importance: It supports immune function, wound healing, and helps maintain taste and smell.

Sources: Meat, dairy products, nuts, seeds, and whole grains.

10. Folate (Vitamin B9):

Importance: It is important for DNA synthesis and red blood cell formation and may help prevent neural tube defects.

Sources: leafy green vegetables, legumes, citrus fruits, and fortified grains.

11. Protein:

Importance: Essential for maintaining muscle mass, supporting immune function, and overall tissue repair.

Sources: Lean meats, poultry, fish, dairy products, eggs, legumes, and plant-based protein sources.

12. Vitamin K:

Importance: supports blood clotting and bone health.

Sources: Leafy green vegetables (kale, spinach, broccoli), cabbage, and Brussels sprouts

13. Antioxidants (Vitamin C, Vitamin E, and Selenium):

Importance: Help protect cells from oxidative stress, supporting overall health.

Sources: Citrus fruits, berries, nuts, seeds, whole grains, and vegetables.

14. Hydration:

Importance: Maintaining proper fluid balance is crucial for overall health, especially as the sense of thirst may decrease with age.

Sources: Water, herbal teas, and hydrating foods like fruits and vegetables.

Role of Nutrition in Managing Endometriosis

The chronic disorder known as endometriosis, which is marked by the growth of tissue resembling the endometrium outside the uterus, is greatly influenced by nutrition. Although diet cannot treat endometriosis on its own, it can have a favorable impact on symptoms, hormone balance, and general health. The following are important facets of how diet plays a part in endometriosis management:

1. Reduction of Inflammation:

Foods that Reduce Inflammation: Endometriosis is characterized by chronic inflammation, which can exacerbate pain and other symptoms. Inflammation can be lessened by eating a diet high in anti-inflammatory foods, such as fruits, vegetables, whole grains, and fatty fish.

2. Endocrine Balance:

Foods That Regulate Hormones: Hormonal balance, particularly the amounts of estrogen that contribute to endometriosis, can be influenced by nutrition. It can be advantageous to eat foods high in phytoestrogens, or estrogen-like chemicals derived from plants, and to enhance hormone metabolism with minerals such as vitamin B6.

3. Balanced Macronutrients: Healthy Fats, Protein, and Carbohydrates:

3. Balanced Macronutrients: Healthy Fats, Protein, and Carbohydrates: An adequate intake of macronutrients supplies the building blocks needed by the body to perform its activities, stabilizes blood sugar, and boosts energy levels. It's critical to include sources of complex carbohydrates, lean protein, and healthy fats.

4. Dietary Fiber:

Fiber for Digestive Health: Fiber promotes regular bowel movements and digestive health. Consuming enough fiber can aid in the management of gastrointestinal symptoms, such as discomfort and bloating, that are frequently linked to endometriosis.

5. Omega-3 Fatty Acids:

Anti-Inflammatory Omega-3s: Rich in walnuts, flaxseeds, chia seeds, and fatty fish, omega-3 fatty acids have anti-inflammatory qualities that may help reduce endometriosis discomfort.

6. Foods Rich in Iron:

Taking on Anemia: Anemia may result from bleeding caused by endometriosis. Eating foods high in iron, such as dark leafy greens, lean meats, and fortified cereals, can help control or prevent anemia.

7. Restricting Trigger Foods:

Determining and Steering Clear of Trigger Foods: Some endometriosis sufferers find relief by knowing which foods to avoid, as these may make their symptoms worse. This can entail cutting back on processed meals, alcohol, and caffeine.

8. Vitamin D and Calcium:

Bone Health: Making sure you're getting enough calcium and vitamin D in your diet is crucial because endometriosis and its therapies can have an influence on bone health. Good sources include dairy products, fortified plant-based milk, and exposure to sunshine.

9. "Staying at a Healthy Weight" and "Controlling Your Weight: Endometriosis management requires maintaining a healthy weight since excess body fat raises estrogen levels. Regular exercise and a well-balanced diet help with weight management.

10. Stress Management:

Mindful Eating and Stress Reduction: Endometriosis symptoms may worsen as a result of ongoing stress. It can be helpful to engage in activities like mindful eating, relaxing techniques, and consuming foods that lower stress.

11. Hydration:

Water's Significance: Maintaining adequate hydration is essential for good health and can ease symptoms like bloating. Proper hydration is facilitated by foods high in water content, herbal teas, and carbohydrates.

12. Personalized Nutrition Plans:

Individualized Approaches: Given that everyone reacts differently to different foods, it's critical to take a customized approach to nutrition. Certain dietary adjustments may provide comfort for some people, so developing a customized plan with a healthcare professional or dietician may be helpful.

CHAPTER FOUR

ANTI-INFLAMMATORY FOODS

Introduction to Anti-Inflammatory Diet

The idea of an anti-inflammatory diet has become well-known as a proactive strategy for wellbeing in a society where chronic inflammation is being acknowledged as a factor in a growing number of health problems. This diet plan emphasizes eating foods with anti-inflammatory qualities in an effort to lessen inflammation in the body and improve general health. Let's investigate the tenets and advantages of the anti-inflammatory diet.

Understanding Inflammation: The body's immunological response naturally includes inflammation, which is why it occurs. On the other hand, persistent inflammation that lasts for a long time can lead to the development of chronic illnesses like diabetes, heart disease, and some types of cancer. To combat this, the anti-inflammatory diet places a focus on foods that have been demonstrated to control the inflammatory response.

The Anti-Inflammatory Diet's Core Elements

1. The Importance of Whole, Plant-Based Foods Whole, nutrient-dense plant foods form the cornerstone of the

anti-inflammatory diet. This includes entire grains, legumes, nuts, seeds, and a range of vibrant fruits and vegetables.

2. Healthy Fats: Inflammation can be significantly reduced by eating healthy fats, especially those high in omega-3 fatty acids. Walnuts, chia seeds, flaxseeds, and fatty fish (such as mackerel and salmon) are some of the sources.

3. Lean Proteins: Prioritize lean protein sources over red and processed meats, such as fish, poultry, lentils, and plant-based proteins. These proteins do not aggravate inflammation while supplying the necessary amino acids.

4. Colorful and antioxidant-rich foods: Antioxidant-rich foods, such as berries, dark leafy greens, and vibrant veggies, help lower inflammation and fight oxidative stress.

5. Whole Grains: Whole grains offer fiber and vital nutrients. Examples of these are brown rice, quinoa, and oats. They contain anti-inflammatory properties and help to maintain stable blood sugar levels.

6. Herbs and Spices: Turmeric, ginger, garlic, and cinnamon are a few examples of herbs and spices that have anti-inflammatory and antioxidant qualities. They are beneficial supplements to the diet that reduce inflammation.

7. Probiotics: Foods that have undergone fermentation, such as kefir, sauerkraut, and yogurt, are rich in probiotics that help maintain gut health. Decreased inflammation is associated with a healthy gut flora.

8. Hydration: An essential component of the anti-inflammatory diet is maintaining adequate hydration. In addition to supporting biological processes, water and another non-sugary beverage help maintain general hydration.

The Anti-Inflammatory Diet's Advantages:

1. Reduced Inflammation: The diet attempts to lessen chronic inflammation in the body by focusing on anti-inflammatory foods and avoiding pro-inflammatory options.

2. Heart Health: Reduced blood pressure and cholesterol are two signs of better cardiovascular health that are linked to an anti-inflammatory diet.

3. Weight control: Placing a focus on whole, nutrient-dense diets may help with healthy weight control by lowering the risk of inflammation associated with obesity.

4. Improved Gut Health: Consuming foods high in probiotics helps maintain a balanced gut microbiota, which is associated with a decrease in inflammation and better digestive health.

5. Joint Health: Adopting an anti-inflammatory diet has been shown to alleviate symptoms in some people with inflammatory joint disorders, such as arthritis.

6. Balanced Blood Sugar Levels: By emphasizing whole grains, fruits, and vegetables, blood sugar levels are kept steady and the inflammation brought on by insulin resistance is decreased.

7. Enhanced Immune Function: Foods high in antioxidants and a diet that is well-balanced support a robust immune system, which aids the body in fighting diseases and infections.

Specific Anti-Inflammatory Foods for Seniors

Seniors can benefit from incorporating specific anti-inflammatory foods into their diets to support overall health and potentially alleviate conditions associated with chronic inflammation. Here are some specific anti-inflammatory foods that can be particularly beneficial for seniors:

1. Fatty Fish:

Examples: Salmon, mackerel, sardines

Why: rich in omega-3 fatty acids, known for their anti-inflammatory properties. These fatty acids can help reduce inflammation and support heart and brain health.

2. Berries:

Examples: blueberries, strawberries, raspberries

Why: Packed with antioxidants, vitamins, and fiber, berries have anti-inflammatory effects and may contribute to cognitive health.

3. Leafy Greens:

Examples: Kale, spinach, Swiss chard

Why: High in vitamins, minerals, and antioxidants, leafy greens provide essential nutrients and have anti-inflammatory properties.

4. Turmeric:

Why: contains curcumin, a potent anti-inflammatory compound. Turmeric has been associated with reduced inflammation and may help manage conditions like arthritis.

5. Broccoli:

Why: A cruciferous vegetable rich in antioxidants and anti-inflammatory compounds, including sulforaphane

6. Nuts and Seeds:

Examples: Walnuts, almonds, chia seeds, flaxseeds

Why: good sources of healthy fats, omega-3 fatty acids, and antioxidants. Nuts and seeds can contribute to heart health and help reduce inflammation.

7. Ginger:

Why: contains gingerol, known for its anti-inflammatory and antioxidant properties. Ginger may help alleviate symptoms of osteoarthritis and may have anti-aging effects.

8. Olive Oil:

Why: Extra virgin olive oil is rich in monounsaturated fats and contains compounds with anti-inflammatory effects. It's a staple in the Mediterranean diet, known for its health benefits.

9. Yogurt:

Why: a source of probiotics that support gut health. A healthy gut microbiome is linked to reduced inflammation and improved overall health.

10. Dark Chocolate:

Why: High-quality dark chocolate with at least 70% cocoa contains flavonoids with anti-inflammatory and antioxidant properties.

11. Green Tea

Why: Rich in polyphenols, green tea has anti-inflammatory and antioxidant effects. It may contribute to cardiovascular health and reduce the risk of chronic diseases.

12. Pineapple:

Why: Contains bromelain, an enzyme with anti-inflammatory properties. Pineapple may help reduce inflammation and promote digestion.

13. Cherries:

Why: Packed with antioxidants and anthocyanins, cherries have anti-inflammatory effects and may be beneficial for managing conditions like gout.

14. Whole Grains:

Examples: Quinoa, brown rice, oats

Why: Whole grains provide fiber and essential nutrients, supporting digestive health and contributing to reduced inflammation.

15. Tomatoes:

Why: Rich in lycopene, tomatoes have antioxidant and anti-inflammatory properties. Cooking tomatoes enhances the availability of lycopene.

Recipes and Meal Ideas

Here's a 2-week anti-inflammatory meal plan with diverse and flavorful recipes. Remember to adjust portion sizes based on individual dietary needs and consult with a healthcare professional or dietitian for personalized advice.

Week 1:

Day 1:

Breakfast: Greek Yogurt Parfait with Berries and Almonds

Lunch: Quinoa Salad with Chickpeas, Cucumber, Tomatoes, and Feta

Dinner: Baked Salmon with Lemon and Dill, Roasted Sweet Potatoes, Steamed Broccoli

Day 2:

Breakfast: Avocado Toast with Poached Egg

Lunch: Lentil and Vegetable Soup

Dinner: Stir-Fried Tofu with Mixed Vegetables, Brown Rice

Day 3:

Breakfast: Smoothie with Spinach, Pineapple, Banana, and Chia Seeds

Lunch: Turkey and Avocado Wrap with Whole Grain Tortilla

Dinner: Grilled Chicken Breast, Quinoa Pilaf, Roasted Brussels Sprouts

Day 4:

Breakfast: Oatmeal with Berries, Walnuts, and a Drizzle of Honey

Lunch: Spinach and Feta Stuffed Bell Peppers

Dinner: Shrimp and Vegetable Stir-Fry, Cauliflower Rice

Day 5:

Breakfast: Whole Grain Pancakes with Fresh Fruit

Lunch: Mediterranean Chickpea Salad

Dinner: Baked Cod with Tomato and Olive Tapenade, Roasted Asparagus

Day 6:

Breakfast: Chia Seed Pudding with Mango and Almond Slices

Lunch: Quinoa and Black Bean Bowl with Avocado

Dinner: Vegetable Curry with Chickpeas and Brown Rice

Day 7:

Breakfast: Smoked Salmon Bagel with Cream Cheese and Capers

Lunch: Kale and Berry Salad with Grilled Chicken

Dinner: Eggplant and Lentil Moussaka

Week 2:

Day 8:

Breakfast: Whole Grain Toast with Almond Butter and Sliced Banana

Lunch: Turkey and Vegetable Stir-Fry with Quinoa

Dinner: Baked Chicken Thighs with Herbs, Roasted Sweet Potatoes, Steamed Green Beans

Day 9:

Breakfast: Berry and Spinach Smoothie Bowl

Lunch: Caprese Salad with Balsamic Glaze, Whole Grain Crackers

Dinner: Grilled Salmon with Mango Salsa, Quinoa Salad

Day 10:

Breakfast: Yogurt Parfait with Granola and Mixed Berries

Lunch: Lentil and Kale Soup

Dinner: Stir-Fried Tofu with Broccoli and Cashews, Brown Rice

Day 11:

Breakfast: Avocado and Tomato Omelet

Lunch: Chickpea and Vegetable Wrap with Hummus

Dinner: Baked Cod with Lemon and Garlic, Roasted Brussels Sprouts, Quinoa

Day 12

Breakfast: Overnight Chia Seed Pudding with Berries

Lunch: Quinoa Salad with Roasted Vegetables and Feta

Dinner: Grilled Chicken Breast, Sweet Potato Mash, Steamed Asparagus

Day 13

Breakfast: Whole Grain Waffles with Greek Yogurt and Mixed Fruit

Lunch: Spinach and Quinoa Stuffed Bell Peppers

Dinner: Shrimp and Vegetable Skewers, Cauliflower Rice

Day 14:

Breakfast: Green Smoothie with Kale, Pineapple, and Banana

Lunch: Turkey and Avocado Salad with Lemon Vinaigrette

Dinner: Eggplant and Chickpea Curry, Brown Rice

CHAPTER FIVE

FOODS TO AVOID

Trigger Foods for Endometriosis

Endometriosis is a disorder in which tissue resembling the lining of the uterus grows outside of it, causing pain, inflammation, and infertility, among other symptoms. Although there isn't a single list of foods that cause endometriosis to flare up, some people say that eating particular foods can make their symptoms worse. It's crucial to remember that each person can have different triggers, and that what works for one person could not work for another. Furthermore, research on the direct relationship between nutrition and endometriosis symptoms is still in its early stages.

Dairy Goods:

Since dairy is thought to increase inflammation, some people with endometriosis decide to limit or avoid dairy. This could apply to yogurt, cheese, and milk.

Foods containing gluten:

Some individuals with endometriosis think about reducing their intake of foods that contain gluten, which is present in wheat and other grains. For certain people, sensitivity to or intolerance to gluten may be a contributing factor to inflammation.

Red Meat:

Consuming a lot of red meat, especially fatty and processed meats, may raise inflammatory levels. Lean protein sources like fish, chicken, or plant-based proteins are preferred by certain people.

Highly Manipulated Foods:

Foods that have been processed and are heavy in harmful fats, artificial additives, and refined sugars may aggravate inflammation. Choosing entire, unprocessed foods is advised frequently.

Coffee:

Caffeine, which is present in coffee, tea, and some sodas, is said by some people to exacerbate their symptoms. It's important to remember that everyone reacts differently to caffeine.

Spirits:

Some people believe that alcohol is an inflammatory substance. Reducing alcohol consumption is an option for those who are controlling their endometriosis symptoms.

Soy-Based Products:

Phytoestrogens are substances derived from plants that have properties similar to those of estrogen and are found in soy. Because of worries about their estrogen levels, some endometriosis sufferers decide to consume fewer soy products.

Foods High in FODMAPs:

A low-FODMAP diet may be used by certain endometriosis sufferers who also have irritable bowel syndrome (IBS) to treat their gastrointestinal symptoms. This diet limits some of the carbs that are present in different foods.

Inflammatory Substances to Limit

Many people find it helpful to limit or stay away from specific drugs that are known to exacerbate inflammatory processes in the body in order to help manage inflammation. Some inflammatory drugs that people might think about restricting are as follows:

1. Red and Processed Meat: Red foods (beef, pork, and lamb) and processed meats (sausages, hot dogs, and the like) may include ingredients that aggravate inflammation. Elevated levels of inflammatory markers are linked to high intake.

2. Refined Sugars: Consuming foods and drinks that include added sugars or refined grains can cause blood sugar levels to jump, which in turn can exacerbate inflammation. These consist of white bread, pastries, sugary drinks, and candies.

3. Saturated and trans fats: Increased inflammation has been linked to trans fats and excessive saturated fats, which are frequently present in baked products, fried foods, and some processed snacks. It is advised to choose healthy fats, such as those found in nuts, avocados, and olive oil.

4. Dairy Items (For Specific Persons): Dairy products have the potential to cause inflammation, and some individuals may be sensitive to them. It's a matter of preference, and people may decide to look into dairy substitutes if they have any suspicions about sensitivity.

5. Highly Processed Foods: Processed foods frequently have harmful fats, artificial additives, and preservatives that can exacerbate inflammation. Generally speaking, choosing whole, minimally processed foods is advised.

6. Overabundance of Omega-6 Fatty Acids: Omega-3 fatty acids, which are included in fish, flaxseeds, and chia seeds, are out of balance and can cause inflammation even though omega-6 fatty acids are necessary. It is recommended to cut back on the consumption of vegetable oils high in omega-6, such as soybean and maize oil.

7. Alcohol: Drinking too much alcohol can cause inflammation throughout the body, especially in the liver. Avoidance or moderation are advised, particularly for those who have medical conditions that make alcohol sensitivity possible.

8. Artificial Additives and Preservatives: Some people may experience inflammatory reactions in response to specific food additives and preservatives. It can be helpful to read food labels and choose foods with fewer additives.

9. Excessive Salt: Consuming a lot of sodium, which is frequently present in restaurant meals and processed foods, can worsen illnesses, including hypertension, and cause inflammation. A better way to control salt intake is to cook at home and choose complete, unprocessed meals.

10. Food Sensitivities: Personal sensitivity to particular foods may be a factor in inflammation. Dairy, gluten, and some allergies are common offenders. Using an elimination diet or allergy testing to identify and steer clear of trigger foods may be beneficial.

11. Coffee (for Certain People): While moderate caffeine consumption is generally thought to be safe, certain people may be sensitive to the drug, and in particular circumstances, excessive caffeine use may exacerbate inflammation.

The Role of Processed Foods in Endometriosis

For people with endometriosis, processed foods may have negative effects because they go through several production steps and frequently include additives, preservatives, and refined substances. There is no one-size-fits-all solution; however, the following factors should be taken into account when examining how processed foods contribute to endometriosis:

1. Inflammation: Processed foods may aggravate inflammation, particularly those heavy in harmful fats, refined sugars, and additives. Reducing inflammatory foods can help manage symptoms, as endometriosis is linked to chronic inflammation.

2. Hormonal Balance: Chemicals and additives included in some processed foods have the potential to throw off the hormonal balance. Because endometriosis is an endocrine disorder, things affecting hormone levels might affect the condition's symptoms.

3. "Deficiency in Certain Nutrients: When comparing processed foods to whole, unprocessed foods, they frequently lack important nutrients. A diet high in nutrients may help people with endometriosis maintain general health and maybe reduce symptoms.

4. Healthy Digestive System: Dietary fiber is essential for gut health but is often lacking in processed diets. A healthy gut flora is supported by enough fiber intake, which also helps reduce constipation, a typical problem for people with endometriosis.

5. Weight Management: Overconsumption and possible weight gain are caused by certain processed foods, which are high in energy but low in nutrients. It's critical to maintain a healthy weight in order to control endometriosis-related symptoms.

6. Insulin Resistance: Diets heavy in added sugars and processed foods can cause insulin resistance, which can affect the balance of hormones. For general health, controlling blood sugar levels with a balanced diet is essential.

7. **Additives Sensitivity:** Some endometriosis sufferers can be sensitive to certain preservatives or additives that are frequently used in processed meals. This sensitivity may show up as gastrointestinal problems or worsen existing symptoms.

8. **Potential for allergies:** Common allergies, including gluten, dairy, and soy, are frequently present in processed meals. An elimination diet that involves identifying and avoiding probable allergens may provide relief for some endometriosis sufferers.

9. **Quality of Fats:** The "fat quality" of the food Unhealthy lipids, including trans fats and high levels of saturated fats, are included in a lot of processed meals. These fats might not promote hormonal balance and might even exacerbate inflammation.

10. **Pre-packaged Convenience vs. Nutrient Density:** Processed foods are popular largely because of their convenience. On the other hand, the body can receive

vital vitamins, minerals, and antioxidants that promote general health by selecting nutrient-dense, whole foods.

CHAPTER SIX

MEAL PLANNING FOR SENIORS

Creating a Personalized Meal Plan

Creating a personalized meal plan involves tailoring your diet to meet your specific nutritional needs, preferences, and health goals. Here's a step-by-step guide to help you create a personalized meal plan:

1. Assess Your Goals and Health Needs:

- **Identify Your Health Goals:** Are you aiming for weight management, improved energy levels, or addressing specific health conditions like endometriosis?

- **Consider Dietary Preferences and Restrictions:** Take note of any food allergies, intolerances, or dietary preferences.

- **Evaluate Your Activity Level:** Your calorie and nutrient needs will depend on your level of physical activity.

2. Determine Your Caloric Needs:

- Use online calculators or consult with a healthcare professional to estimate your daily calorie requirements based on factors like age, gender, weight, and activity level.

3. Plan balanced meals:

- **Include Lean Proteins:** Incorporate sources such as poultry, fish, lean meats, eggs, dairy, legumes, and plant-based proteins.

- **Incorporate Whole Grains:** Choose options like brown rice, quinoa, whole wheat, oats, and barley for fiber and essential nutrients.

- **Include a Variety of Vegetables:** Aim for a colorful mix of vegetables to ensure a broad range of nutrients.

- **Incorporate Healthy Fats:** Include sources like avocados, nuts, seeds, olive oil, and fatty fish for omega-3 fatty acids.

4. Consider Specific Dietary Needs:

For Endometriosis:

- Consider an anti-inflammatory diet with foods rich in omega-3 fatty acids, antioxidants, and whole, unprocessed foods.

- Limit or avoid potential trigger foods such as dairy, gluten, and processed sugars.

For Weight Management:

- Focus on portion control and choose nutrient-dense, whole foods.
- Include a balance of macronutrients (protein, carbohydrates, and fats).

For Specific Health Conditions:

- Consult with a healthcare professional or dietitian to address any dietary restrictions or specific needs related to health conditions.

5. Plan Snacks:

- Choose healthy snacks such as fruits, nuts, yogurt, veggies with hummus, or whole-grain crackers with cheese.

6. Hydration:

- Ensure you stay adequately hydrated with water, herbal teas, and other low-calorie beverages.

7. Consider meal timing:

- Aim for regular, balanced meals throughout the day to maintain energy levels.
- Include pre- and post-workout nutrition if you have an active lifestyle.

8. Meal Prepping:

- Consider batch cooking or meal prepping to make healthy choices more convenient.

9. Listen to Your Body:

- Pay attention to hunger and fullness cues.
- Adjust your meal plan based on how your body responds.

10. Seek professional guidance:

- If you have specific health concerns or conditions, consult with a registered dietitian or healthcare professional for personalized advice.

Sample Day:

Breakfast:

- Scrambled eggs with spinach and tomatoes
- Whole-grain toast
- Fresh berries

Lunch:

- Grilled chicken or tofu salad with mixed greens, cherry tomatoes, cucumbers, and a vinaigrette dressing

- Quinoa or brown rice on the side

Snack:

- Greek yogurt with a handful of almonds

Dinner:

- Baked salmon or lentil curry
- Steamed broccoli and quinoa
- Snack:
- Sliced apple with peanut butter

Weekly Menu Ideas

Here are some weekly menu ideas that incorporate a variety of nutrient-dense foods. These menus are flexible, so feel free to adjust portion sizes and ingredients based on your preferences and dietary needs.

Week 1:

Monday:

Breakfast: Greek yogurt parfait with granola and mixed berries.

Lunch: Quinoa salad with chickpeas, cherry tomatoes, cucumbers, and feta.

Dinner: Grilled chicken breast, sweet potato wedges, and steamed broccoli

Tuesday:

Breakfast: oatmeal with sliced bananas and a sprinkle of chia seeds.

Lunch: Turkey and avocado wrap with a whole-grain tortilla.

Dinner: baked salmon, quinoa pilaf, and roasted Brussels sprouts.

Wednesday:

Breakfast: Smoothie with spinach, pineapple, banana, and Greek yogurt.

Lunch: lentil and vegetable soup.

Dinner: Stir-fried tofu with mixed vegetables served over brown rice.

Thursday:

Breakfast: whole-grain toast with avocado and poached egg.

Lunch: Caprese salad with balsamic glaze and whole-grain crackers.

Dinner: Shrimp and vegetable skewers, quinoa, and a side of mixed greens

Friday:

Breakfast: whole-grain pancakes with fresh berries.

Lunch: Chickpea and vegetable stir-fry with quinoa.

Dinner: Baked cod with lemon and garlic, steamed asparagus, and quinoa

Saturday:

Breakfast: scrambled eggs with sautéed spinach and cherry tomatoes.

Lunch: Mediterranean chickpea salad.

Dinner: Grilled chicken Caesar salad with whole-grain croutons

Sunday:

Breakfast: Chia seed pudding with mango and almond slices.

Lunch: spinach and feta-stuffed bell peppers.

Dinner: Vegetable curry with chickpeas served over brown rice.

Week 2:

Monday:

Breakfast: whole-grain waffles with Greek yogurt and mixed fruit.

Lunch: Turkey and vegetable stir-fry with quinoa.

Dinner: Baked chicken thighs with herbs, roasted sweet potatoes, and steamed green beans

Tuesday:

Breakfast: avocado and tomato omelet.

Lunch: Spinach and quinoa-stuffed bell peppers

Dinner: Grilled salmon with mango salsa and quinoa salad

Wednesday:

Breakfast: overnight oats with almond butter and sliced bananas.

Lunch: Quinoa salad with roasted vegetables and feta.

Dinner: Grilled chicken breast, sweet potato mash, and steamed asparagus

Thursday:

Breakfast: whole-grain toast with almond butter and berries.

Lunch: lentil and kale soup.

Dinner: Stir-fried tofu with broccoli and cashews, brown rice

Friday:

Breakfast: Greek yogurt with honey, walnuts, and a sprinkle of cinnamon.

Lunch: Caprese sandwich with whole grain bread.

Dinner: baked cod with tomato and olive tapenade, roasted Brussels sprouts, and quinoa.

Saturday:

Breakfast: Smoothie bowl with kale, pineapple, and banana.

Lunch: Quinoa and black bean bowl with avocado.

Dinner: eggplant and lentil moussaka.

Sunday:

Breakfast: Smoked salmon bagel with cream cheese and capers

s Kale and berry salad with grilled chicken.

Dinner: eggplant and chickpea curry, served with brown rice.

Tips for Successful Meal Preparation

Meal prep, sometimes referred to as meal preparation, is a fantastic time-saving tactic for managing your nutritional objectives and eating a nutritious diet. The following advice can help you successfully prepare meals:

1. Schedule Meals: Make a weekly or biweekly schedule for your meals. Think about the number of meals and snacks you'll need, as well as your dietary preferences and nutritional requirements.

2. Select balanced dishes: Look for dishes that have an appropriate ratio of whole grains, fruits, vegetables, lean proteins, and healthy fats. This guarantees a wholesome, well-balanced diet.

3. Batch Cooking: Make big quantities of essential components, such as roasted veggies, cereals, and meats. This simplifies the process of putting together meals for the week.

4. Invest in Storage Containers: To keep your ready goods and meals organized, use a variety of storage containers. For convenience, think about using microwaveable and dishwasher-safe containers.

5. Portion Control: To prevent overindulging and to have meals ready to go throughout the week, portion meals out into individual containers.

6. Label and Date: Write the contents and the preparation date on the labels of your containers. This keeps food waste at bay and makes it easier to monitor freshness.

7. Prepare Snacks: Cut up vegetables, cut up fruit, or portion out nuts as healthy snacks. Having these close at hand can help you avoid reaching for less healthy choices.

8. Take Freezing into Account: Certain dishes and components work nicely frozen. If you have additional time one day, think about preparing extra portions and freezing them.

9. Use versatile items: To add diversity without requiring a long list of items, select ingredients that may be utilized in several different meals.

10. Keep Your Kitchen Organized: Make sure your kitchen is kept tidy. Organize the components anyway you see fit, and make sure that frequently used goods are always close at hand.

11. Set Aside Time: Plan a certain period of time every week to prepare meals. Making meal preparation a sustainable habit requires consistency.

CHAPTER SEVEN

HORMONE-BALANCING FOODS

Understanding Hormones and Endometriosis

To fully appreciate the complexity of endometriosis, one must grasp the connection between hormones and the medical disease. Since endometriosis is an estrogen-dependent condition, its onset and course are significantly influenced by the presence and activity of estrogen.

1. The Regular Menstrual Cycle: During the follicular phase of a typical menstrual cycle, which occurs prior to ovulation, an increase in estrogen levels causes the endometrial lining to thicken in anticipation of a possible pregnancy. Progesterone levels rise following ovulation in order to maintain the endometrial lining and prime the body for a fertilized egg. In the event that pregnancy is not achieved, a decrease in estrogen and progesterone levels causes the endometrial lining to shed during the menstrual cycle.

2. The Function of Estrogen: The main source of estrogen is the ovaries, and it is essential for maintaining the female reproductive system and controlling the menstrual cycle. Progesterone and estrogen levels are out of balance in endometriosis, with estrogen dominance being a prevalent characteristic. The aberrant development of tissue outside the uterus that resembles endometrial tissue is a result of this imbalance.

3. Tissue Outside the Uterus: That Is Similar to Endometrial: Tissue that resembles the endometrium, or the lining of the uterus, develops outside the uterus in endometriosis. This tissue reacts to changes in hormones in a manner akin to that of the uterine lining and is referred to as endometriotic lesions or implants. These lesions change as well, growing, inflaming, and bleeding during the menstrual cycle as estrogen levels rise and fall.

4. Inflammation and Pain: The pelvic region may experience inflammation, scarring, and adhesion formation as a result of endometriotic lesions. Particularly during menstruation (dysmenorrhea), sexual activity (dyspareunia), and other activities, this may cause pain.

5. Estrogen Sensitivity: Endometriotic lesions frequently have estrogen receptors expressed on them, which makes them susceptible to the body's estrogen levels. Elevated amounts of estrogen may promote the development and activity of these lesions.

6. Impact on Fertility: Endometriosis can have an impact on fertility, and the disorder's hormonal imbalances can exacerbate infertility.

7. Hormonal Treatments: Endometriosis is frequently managed with hormonal medications that work to control estrogen levels. These could include aromatase inhibitors, gonadotropin-releasing hormone (GnRH) agonists, and hormonal contraceptives.

8. Menopausal Transition: For those with endometriosis, the menopause, which is marked by the normal decrease in reproductive hormones, frequently results in symptom relief. Nonetheless, in certain instances, the ailment may endure, and indications may fluctuate throughout the menopause.

Foods that Support Hormonal Balance

Maintaining hormonal balance is crucial for overall health, and certain foods can contribute to hormonal equilibrium. While diet alone cannot entirely regulate hormonal levels, incorporating nutrient-dense foods may support hormonal balance. Here are some foods that are generally considered supportive:

1. Fatty Fish:

Examples: Salmon, mackerel, trout

Why: rich in omega-3 fatty acids, which can help reduce inflammation and support hormone production.

2. Avocados:

Why: High in monounsaturated fats, avocados provide a healthy source of energy and support hormone production.

3. Nuts and Seeds:

Examples: walnuts, almonds, flaxseeds, and chia seeds.

Why: Rich in healthy fats, fiber, and antioxidants, nuts and seeds contribute to overall health and may support hormonal balance.

4. Leafy Greens:

Examples: Kale, spinach, Swiss chard

Why: Packed with vitamins, minerals, and antioxidants, leafy greens support overall health and may contribute to hormonal balance.

5. Cruciferous Vegetables:

Examples: broccoli, cauliflower, and Brussels sprouts.

Why: contain compounds like indole-3-carbinol that may help balance estrogen levels in the body.

6. Berries:

Examples: blueberries, strawberries, raspberries

Why: Rich in antioxidants and fiber, berries support overall health and may have anti-inflammatory effects.

7. Greek Yogurt:

 Why: A source of protein and probiotics, Greek yogurt supports gut health, which is linked to hormonal balance.

8. Quinoa:

Why: whole grain that provides complex carbohydrates, fiber, and essential nutrients, supporting overall health.

9. Fermented Foods:

Examples: Kimchi, sauerkraut, yogurt

Why: Rich in probiotics that promote gut health, which is linked to hormonal regulation,

10. Wild-caught salmon:

Why: high in omega-3 fatty acids, vitamin D, and protein, supporting overall health and hormonal balance.

11. Sweet Potatoes:

Why: A good source of complex carbohydrates, fiber, and beta-carotene, sweet potatoes provide steady energy.

12. Turmeric:

Why: contains curcumin, which has anti-inflammatory properties and may support hormonal balance.

13. Green Tea:

Why: Rich in antioxidants, green tea may have positive effects on hormonal health.

14. Legumes:

Examples: lentils, chickpeas, and black beans.

Why: Provide plant-based protein, fiber, and various nutrients that support overall health.

15. Eggs:

Why: Eggs, a good source of high-quality protein and various nutrients, support overall health.

Incorporating Hormone-Balancing Foods into the Diet

Incorporating hormone-balancing foods into your diet involves making conscious choices to include nutrient-dense options that may positively influence hormonal health. Here's a guide on how to integrate these foods into your meals:

1. Fatty Fish:

Incorporate into your diet: Aim for at least two servings of fatty fish per week. Grill, bake, or steam salmon, mackerel, or trout.

2. Avocados:

Incorporate into your diet: Add sliced avocados to salads and smoothies, or enjoy them on whole-grain toast.

3. Nuts and Seeds:

Incorporate into your diet: Snack on a handful of nuts or seeds, sprinkle them on yogurt, or add them to salads.

4. Leafy Greens:

Incorporate into your diet: Make salads with a mix of kale, spinach, and Swiss chard. Add leafy greens to smoothies, or sauté them as a side dish.

5. Cruciferous Vegetables:

Incorporate into your diet: Steam or stir-fry broccoli, cauliflower, and Brussels sprouts. Include them in salads or as a side dish.

6. Berries:

Incorporate into your diet: Enjoy berries as a snack, add them to yogurt, or blend them into smoothies.

7. Greek Yogurt:

Incorporate into your diet: Use Greek yogurt as a base for parfaits and smoothie bowls, or enjoy it as a snack with a drizzle of honey.

8. Quinoa:

Incorporate into your diet: Use quinoa as a base for salads, mix it into soups, or serve it as a side dish with grilled vegetables.

9. Fermented Foods:

Incorporate into your diet: Include fermented foods like kimchi, sauerkraut, or yogurt as a side dish or snack.

10. Wild-Caught Salmon:

Incorporate into your diet: Grill or bake wild-caught salmon and pair it with a side of steamed vegetables or quinoa.

11. Sweet Potatoes:

Incorporate into your diet: Roast sweet potatoes as a side dish, mash them, or add them to salads.

12. Turmeric:

Incorporate into your diet: Use turmeric in cooking, such as in curries, soups, or as a spice for roasted vegetables.

13. Green Tea:

Incorporate into your diet: Swap out sugary beverages for green tea. Enjoy it, hot or cold.

14. Legumes:

Incorporate into your diet: Include lentils, chickpeas, or black beans in salads, soups, or as a protein source in main dishes.

15. Eggs:

Incorporate into your diet: Prepare eggs in various ways—boiled, poached, scrambled, or as omelets.

Tips for Incorporating These Foods:

1. Meal Prepping: Plan your meals in advance, incorporating a variety of these foods to ensure a balanced and nutritious diet.

2. Smoothies: Blend hormone-balancing foods like berries, leafy greens, and seeds into delicious smoothies.

3. Snacking Smart: Choose nuts, seeds, or Greek yogurt as healthy snacks.

4. Diverse Recipes: Experiment with new recipes that feature these foods in creative ways.

5. Mindful Eating: Pay attention to portion sizes and listen to your body's hunger and fullness cues.

CHAPTER EIGHT

MINDFUL EATING FOR ENDOMETRIOSIS

The Connection Between Stress and Endometriosis

Endometriosis and stress have a complicated and multidimensional relationship. Although endometriosis is not caused by stress per se, there is evidence that stress may contribute to the onset and aggravation of endometriosis symptoms.

1. The Effect on Symptoms: Although stress doesn't directly cause endometriosis, it can make symptoms worse. Stress can make endometriosis symptoms worse, including pain, exhaustion, and other symptoms.

2. Hormonal Influence: The equilibrium of hormones can be affected by stress. Endometriosis-related reproductive hormones, progesterone and estrogen, may be impacted by the release of stress hormones like cortisol.

3. Immune System Response: Stress has an impact on the immune system, which may have an impact on the body's capacity to control and minimize inflammatory reactions. Inflammation is a hallmark of endometriosis, and stress may exacerbate this inflammatory milieu.

4. Perception of Pain: Stress can intensify one's experience of pain. Stressful situations may cause endometriosis sufferers to become more sensitive to pain.

5. Effect on the Menstrual Cycle: Period regularity may be impacted by menstrual cycle disruption caused by stress. Given that endometriosis is linked to hormone swings, this may be important for those who have the condition.

6. Life Quality: It can be difficult to manage a chronic illness like endometriosis on your own. Chronic stress can be caused by difficulties managing symptoms, issues with fertility, and the effects on day-to-day functioning.

7. Partnership in Both Directions: It's critical to understand that endometriosis and stress have a reciprocal relationship. Stress can aggravate symptoms associated with endometriosis, thus starting a vicious cycle in which stress exacerbates symptoms and symptoms exacerbate stress.

8. Mechanisms of Coping: Stress can cause people to develop coping mechanisms, and these coping mechanisms can affect lifestyle choices, including food, exercise, and sleep. These lifestyle choices may, therefore, have an impact on how endometriosis is managed.

9. Mind-Body Practices: Mind-body techniques like yoga, meditation, and deep breathing exercises can help people with endometriosis manage their stress and, in some situations, enhance their general wellbeing.

10. Single-person Variability: The effects of stress on endometriosis can differ greatly from person to person. Some people may discover that stress has a major impact on their symptoms, while others might not see a discernible relationship.

Mindful Eating Techniques

Savoring each bite, being in the present, and giving the eating experience your whole attention are all parts of mindful eating. To foster a more aware relationship with food, consider these 15 mindful eating practices:

1. Eat Distraction-Free: Switch off electronics, store books, and concentrate only on the act of eating. Distractions must be removed in order for you to fully enjoy the tastes and textures of your food.

2. Activate Your Senses: Take note of your food's hues, textures, and scents. Before you take a mouthful, take some time to enjoy the flavors and sights of your meal.

3. "Chew Slowly: Give your food a good chewing motion and enjoy every taste. Take note of the texture and flavor. Slow chewing facilitates digestion as well.

4. Set Your Cutlery Down: Take pauses throughout your meal to set down your cutlery. This gives you the opportunity to stop, take a breath, and pay attention to your body's signals of hunger and fullness.

5. Thank You Expression: Give some thought to your thanks for the meal that is in front of you before you start eating. Think back on its origins and the work that went into getting it ready.

6. Listen to Your Body: Be aware of your body's signals of hunger and fullness. Consume food only when you're hungry, and quit when you're full. Learn to listen to your body's signals and avoid overindulging.

7. Mindful Portioning: Give yourself sensible serving sizes to prevent thoughtless overindulgence in food. In the event that you become more hungry, you can always return.

8. Take Small Bites: Take smaller, more deliberate bites as opposed to larger ones. This gives you a more complete experience of the flavors and textures.

9. Interval Between Bits: In between bites, set down your utensils. You can take a moment to taste the taste again and gauge how hungry you are.

10. Check in with Emotions: Pay attention to how you're feeling both before and after meals. Refrain from utilizing food as a coping mechanism for emotions or stress.

11. Eat with All Your Senses: During your meal, use every sensation. Savor the flavors, listen to the noises, feel the textures, and smell the fragrances.

12. Conscious Inhalation: Breathe deeply both before and during your meal. This encourages relaxation and assists in bringing your attention to the here and now.

13. "Savor Every Meal: Take a moment to savor the tastes and experiences after every meal. By doing this, you can learn to slow down and savor your meal.

14. Express Gratitude After the Meal: Once your meal is finished, give thanks to your body for the food it got. Consider the advantages of the dining experience.

15. Use Mindful Eating Apps or Guides: To help you establish and sustain mindfulness practices around food, make use of apps or guided mindful eating exercises. These resources are able to offer organized assistance.

Relaxation and Stress Reduction Strategies for Seniors

In particular for seniors, relaxation and stress management are critical elements of general wellbeing. Seniors can employ the following measures to improve relaxation and reduce stress in their everyday routines:

1. Deep Breathing Exercises: To soothe the nervous system, engage in deep breathing exercises. Take a deep breath via your nose, hold it for a little while, and then gently release it through your mouth.

2. Mindfulness Meditation: To stay present and lower stress, practice mindfulness meditation. Pay attention to your breathing, your body's feelings, or your surroundings.

3. Progressive Muscle Relaxation (PMR): Tense each muscle group, working your way up to your head, and then gradually relax it. This method encourages both mental and physical relaxation.

4. Guided Imagery: Contemplate serene settings or envision successful results by employing guided imagery. By doing so, the emphasis might be diverted from stressors.

5. Yoga: Mild yoga postures and stretches improve balance, flexibility, and calmness. A lot of courses and online tools are designed with elders in mind.

6. Tai Chi: Combining soft movements and deep breathing, Tai Chi is a low-impact workout. It encourages flexibility, balance, and relaxation.

7. Aromatherapy: Use scented candles, diffusers, or essential oils to create a tranquil atmosphere with aromas like lavender or chamomile.

8. Massage Therapy: To ease tension and relax muscles, think about getting regular massages or practicing self-massage.

9. Listening to Music: Take pleasure in soothing sounds or music. Make playlists with your favorite songs or listen to music from genres that are thought to promote calm.

10. Nature Walks: Take leisurely strolls in a park or garden to spend time in nature. Both the body and the mind can find calmness in nature.

11. Reading: Immerse yourself in a well-written book or do some light reading. Through reading, one can escape tension and enter other worlds.

12. Social Connection: Continue to have social relationships with loved ones. Positive encounters can lessen feelings of loneliness and offer emotional support.

13. Art and Creativity: Take part in artistic endeavors like crafts, painting, or drawing. Artistic self-expression has therapeutic benefits.

14. Warm Baths: Take warm baths scented with relaxing oils, such as eucalyptus or lavender. Muscles can be relaxed, and the mind can be calmed by warm water.

15. Laughter Therapy: See a humorous film, go to a comedy show, or hang out with amusing people. Laughter is good for your body and mind in many ways.

16. Journaling: Record your feelings and ideas in a notebook. This can aid with emotional processing and clarity-seeking.

17. Sleeping techniques: Before going to bed, engage in soothing breathing techniques to encourage relaxation and enhance the quality of your sleep.

CHAPTER NINE

LIFESTYLE HABITS FOR LONG-TERM MANAGEMENT

Regular Physical Activity for Seniors with Endometriosis

It is imperative that seniors, even those who have endometriosis, engage in regular physical activity. Numerous advantages can come from exercising, such as better mood, more strength and flexibility, and general health improvements. But it's important to approach exercise with awareness of certain medical issues, such as endometriosis.

1. Consult with Healthcare Professionals: Speak with your primary care physician or gynecologist as well as the rest of your healthcare team prior to beginning any workout regimen. Depending on your unique health situation and the intensity of your endometriosis symptoms, they can offer advice.

2. Low-Impact Cardiovascular Exercise: Take part in cardiovascular exercises that have a low impact on the pelvic region and are easy on the joints. Walking, swimming, stationary cycling, and elliptical exercise are among the available options.

3. Strength Training: To preserve bone density and muscular mass, include strength training activities. For resistance, use resistance bands or light weights. Pay attention to exercises that work the main muscle groups.

4. Stretching and Flexibility: To increase range of motion and lessen stiffness, use stretching and flexibility exercises. Stretching exercises and yoga can be helpful. Select stretches and poses that your body feels comfortable doing.

5. Mind-Body Practices: Take into account mind-body exercises like qigong or tai chi. These exercises are well recognized for fostering balance and relaxation because they combine deep breathing with soft movements.

6. Exercises on the Pelvic Floor: Exercises on the Pelvic Floor, such as Kegel exercises, can help strengthen the pelvic muscles. Seek advice on suitable exercises from a physical therapist or other medical expert.

7. Change the Duration and Intensity: Observe your body's cues and adjust the amount of time and intensity of your workouts according to how you feel. Refrain from exerting excessive force on yourself, particularly when experiencing more pain or discomfort.

8. **Remain Hydrated:** It's critical to stay well-hydrated, particularly when exercising. To maintain general health and stay hydrated, regularly consume water.

9. **Listen to Your Body:** Pay attention to how your body reacts to physical activity. Consult your healthcare physician and adjust or cease the exercise if you feel more pain or discomfort.

10. **Warm-Up and Cool-Down:** Make sure your workout regimen always includes a suitable warm-up and cool-down. This promotes healing and gets your body ready for exercise.

11. **Select Activities You Enjoy:** To make exercise more pleasurable and long-lasting, choose activities you enjoy. Finding activities, you love to do, whether it's dancing, gardening, or sports, enhances the chances that you'll remain with them.

12. **Regular Check-Ins:** Talk about your exercise regimen and any changes in symptoms with your healthcare physician on a regular basis. This guarantees that your overall health goals and your physical activity strategy are in sync.

Importance of Hydration

Staying well hydrated is essential for preserving general health and wellbeing. The following 15–20 points emphasize how crucial it is to stay hydrated:

1. Cellular Function: Water supports and facilitates nutrient transfer, which is necessary for the correct operation of cells.

2. Temperature Regulation: Through activities like sweating and heat dissipation, adequate hydration aids in the regulation of body temperature.

3. Joint Lubrication: Water helps lubricate joints, promoting easy mobility and lowering the incidence of joint discomfort.

4. Cognitive Function: Drinking enough water helps with focus, attentiveness, and short-term memory, among other cognitive functions.

5. Digestive Health: Water is essential for nutrient absorption and digestion. It promotes a healthy digestive tract and aids in the prevention of constipation.

6. Nutrient Transport: Water acts as a conduit for nutrients to go throughout the body, supplying vital elements to tissues and cells.

7. Heart Health: Maintaining blood volume and enhancing the heart's ability to pump blood more effectively are two benefits of proper hydration that promote cardiovascular health.

8. Kidney Function: To support the generation of urine and the filtering of waste products, an adequate intake of water is necessary for healthy kidney function.

9. Skin Health: Hydration encourages skin elasticity and contributes to the preservation of a clear complexion. Dehydration may be a factor in dryness and early aging.

10. Weight Management: By encouraging a sensation of fullness, drinking water before meals can help regulate appetite and promote weight management.

11. Electrolyte Balance: Adequate hydration maintains the balance of electrolytes, which are necessary for a number of body processes. This is especially crucial in hot conditions and when engaging in vigorous exercise.

12. Muscle Function: Staying hydrated is essential to preserving muscle tone and avoiding cramping when exercising.

13. Detoxification: Water supports the body's detoxification processes by assisting the urine's ability to rid the body of waste and pollutants.

14. Immune System Support: A strong immune system, which aids in the body's defense against infections and illnesses, is linked to proper hydration.

15. Decrease in weariness: Low energy and weariness are two effects of dehydration. Maintaining hydration can boost general energy levels and help fight fatigue.

16. Headache Prevention: One common cause of headaches and migraines is dehydration. Keeping your hydration intake appropriate can help avoid these symptoms.

17. Enhanced Exercise Outcomes: Adequate hydration is crucial for peak sports performance, bolstering stamina, power, and recuperation both during and after physical activity.

18. Blood Pressure Regulation: Maintaining blood volume and supporting blood pressure regulation are two benefits of proper hydration.

19. Avoiding Heat-Related Illnesses: It's essential to stay hydrated in hot weather and when engaging in vigorous physical exercise to avoid heat-related disorders like heatstroke.

20. Emotional State and Mood: Maintaining adequate hydration promotes mental clarity and emotional wellbeing. Dehydration can have an adverse effect on mood and cognitive performance.

Sleep and Its Impact on Endometriosis Symptoms

Sleep is an essential component of good health and can have a big impact on a lot of different parts of life, including endometriosis symptoms. Sleep can affect endometriosis symptoms in the following ways:

1. Feeling of Pain: A good night's sleep is associated with a decreased feeling of pain. Resting enough can help control the pain that comes with endometriosis, which can include pain during sexual activity, pelvic pain, and dysmenorrhea (menstrual cramps).

2. Inflammation: Sleep is necessary for controlling the body's inflammation. One of the main characteristics of endometriosis is chronic inflammation, which can be exacerbated by inadequate sleep.

3. Endocrine Control: Hormone balance is influenced by sleep, and sleep disturbances can impact the levels of estrogen and progesterone, for example. The symptoms of endometriosis are linked to variations in hormone levels.

4. Immune Function: A robust immune system is supported by getting enough sleep. For those who already have endometriosis, this is especially important because immune system malfunction may contribute to the onset and course of the disease.

5. Mood and Mental Health: Sleep has an impact on both mental and emotional well-being. Being emotionally impacted by having endometriosis can be made worse by poor sleep quality, which is linked to elevated levels of stress, anxiety, and sadness.

6. Weariness: Pain and inflammation, along with endometriosis symptoms, can all lead to weariness. Getting enough sleep is crucial for controlling fatigue and boosting vitality in general.

7. Inconsistencies in Menstruation: The circadian clock can be upset by irregular sleep patterns or insufficient sleep, which may have an effect on menstrual regularity. Hormonal abnormalities associated with sleep disturbances may impact endometriosis symptoms.

8. Quality of Life: Sleep disorders that persist over time can have a detrimental effect on general quality of life. When sleep is addressed, endometriosis patients may see improvements in their overall health and day-to-day functioning.

Strategies for Enhanced Sleep in Endometriosis Patients:

1. Make a regular sleep schedule: To help your body's internal clock function properly, go to bed and wake up at the same time every day.

2. Establish a Calm Bedtime Routine: Before going to bed, try some relaxing exercises like light stretching, reading, or meditation to let your body know its time to unwind.

3. Maximize Your Sleep Environment: Make sure your bedroom is a restful place to be. Maintain the space cool, quiet, and dark. Invest in pillows and a comfy mattress.

4. Limit stimulants: cut back on or completely stop using caffeine and nicotine in the hours before bed.

5. Manage Stress: To encourage relaxation before bed, engage in stress-relieving activities like mindfulness meditation or deep breathing exercises.

6. Limit Screen Time: Refrain from using electronics for at least one hour before going to bed. The melatonin generation of the sleep hormone may be disrupted by the blue light emitted from displays.

7. Regular Exercise: Move around often, but try to avoid doing a lot of strenuous exercise right before bed.

8. Seek Professional Help: If sleep issues continue, think about speaking with a medical expert or sleep specialist for an additional assessment and direction.

CONCLUSION

In summary, the complex relationship between sleep and endometriosis highlights an important—yet frequently overlooked—aspect of treating this difficult condition. Sleep affects endometriosis symptoms in more ways than just relaxation and recuperation; it also affects inflammation, hormone balance, pain perception, and general wellbeing.

Good sleep is a powerful pain-sensing mechanism that may help endometriosis sufferers cope with the often-crippling pelvic pain, dysmenorrhea, and discomfort that come with the disease. Additionally, since persistent inflammation is a defining feature of endometriosis and a contributor in its progression, sleep's function in controlling inflammation assumes important.

The fine dance of hormones, such as progesterone and estrogen, is closely related to endometriosis symptoms and sleep habits. Sleep disturbances have the ability to upset the hormonal balance and exacerbate the endometriosis-related hormonal abnormalities. Furthermore, good sleep is essential for the immune system, which is another important endometriosis component, to function at its best. This suggests that endometriosis patients may benefit from boosting their immune responses.

Sleep is a key factor in mood, mental health, and fatigue—all of which are frequently impacted in endometriosis sufferers. Since sleep and mental health are inversely correlated, treating sleep disorders is crucial to treating the emotional toll that having endometriosis has on a person's life.

It is crucial for those managing the complications of endometriosis to implement techniques that enhance their quality of sleep. Crucial to promoting improved sleep hygiene include setting up regular sleep patterns, establishing calming nighttime rituals, improving sleep settings, and reducing stress. Comprehensive care also includes acknowledging the special difficulties associated with endometriosis and designing interventions that put the patient's physical and mental health first.

Essentially, putting a high priority on getting enough sleep shows up as a potent tool in the holistic approach to managing endometriosis as well as a way to obtain restful sleep. The correlation shown between sleep deprivation and symptoms of endometriosis highlights the significance of including sleep hygiene within the wider range of healthcare interventions. This could provide individuals with an opportunity to improve their overall well-being, quality of life, and ability to control their symptoms. In order to provide endometriosis patients with comprehensive care, treating sleep disruptions is expected to become increasingly important as scientific awareness of this relationship advances.